Home Remedies

For Colds

Fever And Sore Throat

Home Remedies

For Colds

Fever And Sore Throat

By Monica Sidoine,

S.N.H.S. Dip. Herbalism

DISCLAIMER

This book is to serve as an informational guide for use in the home. The remedies and procedures contained in this book are meant to supplement and are not intended to be a substitute for professional medical care. Please seek a qualified medical practitioner for all ailments. The author nor distributors takes no responsibility for customers choosing to treat themselves. Your use of this information is at your own risk.

ISBN - 13: 978-1534832930
ISBN - 10: 1534832939

Proof Read by Jasmine Ned Anunda

Printed By Create Space Publishing
United States of America

ACKNOWLEDGMENTS

I would like to thank all those who have contributed in one way or another to the completion of HOME REMEDIES FOR COLDS, FEVER AND SORE THROAT.

I thank God for giving me the vision, wisdom and good health to write this book. For all he has done and will continue to do in my life.

For the many prayer warriors who interceded on behalf of this project and also their moral support.

I thank my daughter Jasmine Ned Anunda for proof reading.

Thank you all.

Monica Sidoine.

PREFACE

The procedures in this Book was designed to be as simple as possible so that anyone will be able to follow them. Most of the items used are local things which you would either have at home, in your kitchen garden or can be easily purchased from the local market or health store for a very low cost.

TABLE OF CONTENTS

COLDS

What is a cold?
A cold is a viral infection of the nose, throat and bronchial tubes.

What are the causes?
The main reason of a cold is a virus, which can enter your
body directly or indirectly through the mouth, nose, or even eyes.
Coughing or sneezing.
Hand shaking.
Not getting enough rest.
The body being exposed to cold weather.
Sharing of contaminated utensils, towels and other objects.

What are the symptoms?
Harsh voice.
Loss of appetite.
Sneezing, coughing, runny nose.
Nasal and chest congestion, headaches, watery eyes, fever, chills.
Muscle aches, mild fatigue, pain.
Temporary loss of taste and smell, bad taste buds.
Sore throat due to chocking and accumulation of cough.
Itching and irritation in the nasal passage.
Clogged ears due to accumulation of cough.

NATURAL REMEDIES

- Boil potato peelings about ½"thick for about 20 minutes. Strain, cool and drink. Make it fresh every day.

- **Garlic Syrup:** Put 1 cup of finely minced garlic, 1 teaspoon powdered cloves and 1 ½ tablespoons grated ginger or 1 teaspoon powdered ginger in a pan. Add enough honey or molasses to cover it. Cover and simmer on low heat for about 25 minutes stirring constantly to avoid burning. A little water can be added.
  Take 1 tablespoon for adults or teenagers, 1 teaspoon for children every hour or as needed.

- **Eucalyptus syrup:** Boil 1oz of dried eucalyptus leaves in 2 cups of water for 10 minutes. Steep for 20 minutes. Strain and add 11oz of honey. Bottle.
  Take 1 teaspoon 3 times daily.

- **Onion syrup:** Boil several thinly sliced or blended onions with some water and plenty of honey or brown sugar.
  Take by tablespoons as needed.

- Blend 1 onion, add 1 glass of lemon, tomato or carrot juice. Have ½ a glass twice daily taken by spoonful's.

- Stir ½ teaspoon powdered turmeric in 1 cup of hot milk, add a pinch of salt, ginger or cayenne.
  Drink 1 cup 3 times daily.

- Blend 1 grapefruit, 1 orange, 2 lemons, 3 garlic cloves and ½ of a large onion with enough water so that the mixture can turn in the blender. Add 3 drops of peppermint oil. Refrigerate.

Warm before serving.
Adults 1 cup daily, children ½ cup, taken by spoonful at a time during the day.

- Blend 2 lemons with some water very well. Add 4 spoonful's of honey and enough water to make 2 liters. Strain.
  Drink it throughout the day.

- Steep 1oz of lemon grass in 1 liter of boiling water for 30 minutes.
  Drink 1 cup 4 times daily.

- Steep 1oz of ginger in 1 liter of boiling water for 20 minutes.
  Drink 1 cup three times daily.

- Steep 4 tablespoons eucalyptus leaves to 2 liters of boiling water for 10 minutes.
  Take 8 cups throughout the day.

- Steep 1oz of basil in 1 liter of boiling water for 30 minutes.
  Take 1 cup 3 times daily.

- Steep 1oz of chamomile in 1 liter of boiling water for 30 minutes.
  Take 1 cup 3 times daily.

- Steep 1oz of red clover in 1 liter of boiling water for 30 minutes.
  Take 1 cup 3 times daily.

- Steep 1oz of patchouli leaves in 1 liter of boiling water for 30 minutes.
  Take 1 cup 3 times daily.

- Steep 10 neem leaves to 4 cups of boiling water for 30 minutes. Take 1 cup 3 times daily.

- Steep 6 avocado leaves in 1 liter of boiling water for 30 minutes.
  Drink 1 cup twice daily.

- Simmer 2 glasses of water along with 1 tablespoon of powdered cinnamon and 2 cloves for 15 minutes. Strain.
  Drink 1 warm cup twice daily.

- Crush 10 garlic cloves and boil it in 3 cups of water for 5 minutes. Strain it and add 2 teaspoons of honey.
  Drink 1 cup twice daily.

- Mix the juice of 1 lime and 1 teaspoon of honey in 1 glass of warm water.
  Take it twice daily, the last one just before bedtime.

- Drink citrus fruit juice during the day.

- Simmer several garlic cloves in a small pan of water for 20 minutes until very soft. Mash the garlic. Add an equal amount of honey, ½ teaspoon cayenne powder and stir in 1 tablespoon lime or lemon juice.
  Take 1 teaspoon every 15 minutes.

- Make a paste with equal amounts of ginger and cloves, add a pinch of salt to it.
  Eat ½ a teaspoon twice daily.

- **Onion broth:** Take 3 large onions and slice thinly, boil into a broth.

Take it 3 times daily.

- **Clove soup:** Combine 1 pint of vegetable stock, 2 onions thinly sliced, 1 bay leaf, 6 cloves and salt to taste. Bring to a boil then simmer for 30 minutes. Remove the bay leaf and cloves. Serve it hot.

- Drink lots of water throughout the day at least 8 – 10 glasses.

- Increase intake of foods high in vitamin C: grapefruit, oranges, lemons, guavas, tomatoes etc.

- Eat 3 raw garlic cloves three times daily with meals.

- Chew some raw ginger.

- **Steam inhalation** – Using any of the following. Inhale for 15 minutes 3 times daily.
  See the Hydrotherapy Section.

  1) 6 drops eucalyptus oil to 1 cup of boiling water, cloves and or thyme.
  2) Vicks vapoRub or wintergreen oil.
  3) Boil 20 neem leaves in 1 quart of water.
  4) Crush 10 garlic cloves in 1 quart of water and simmer for 15 minutes.
  5) Put 1 drop of basil oil in a bowl of hot water.
  6) 5 drops of lavender essential oil in 1 quart of water.

- Dilute the juice of one onion in water.
  Taken in drops through the nostrils.

- Mix ½ teaspoon blended garlic, 32oz water and the juice of 1 onion together.
  Take 25 drops every 4 hours by mouth and nostrils.

- Add 1 teaspoon salt to a pint of warm water, sniff it up the nose then blow it out gently. Repeat until the nose is entirely clean of mucous.
  Then gargle the throat and rinse the mouth out thoroughly with 1 glass of warm water to ½ teaspoon salt three times daily. Take a hot shower after.
  This treatment will keep the nose and mouth clean preventing the cold from going down into the lungs.
  //

- Blow your nose regularly. Hold one nostril while blowing mucus from the other and then switch to the other.

- Sprinkle a few drops of menthol on the pillow to inhale it.

- Sauté some minced onion and add 1 cup of vinegar in it.
  Then add some cornmeal to make a thick paste. Put the paste in a muslin cloth and cover it.
  Apply it on your chest and throat area.
  Cover with a blanket or towel.
  Leave it on for 15 minutes.

- Hot Sweat Bath

- Hot Foot Bath.
  See the Hydrotherapy Section for Hot Sweat and Hot Foot Bath.

Health Tips

- Always wash your hands before touching eyes, nose and mouth.

- Use paper towels to dry your hands and throw them away after use.

- Go to bed early and try to get at least eight hours of rest.

- Elevate the head a little more when ready to sleep.

- Take walks daily for at least half an hour while inhaling the fresh air.

- While sneezing, cover your face with a handkerchief.

- Always clear and clean stuffy nose.

- Always keep surroundings clean.

- Maintain a healthy lifestyle.

- Try to control your stress to avoid your immune system from getting weak.

- Avoid getting close to persons if you or they have a cold.

- Avoid smoking, especially during the period of your cold.

- Avoid sugar and excess fat.

- Don't share utensils and towels with the infected person.

FEVER

What is a Fever?
A fever is a body temperature that is unusually high above the normal range. It is basically a symptom of another condition or illness. It can occur when your body is fighting an infection, such as the flu. It helps to destroy the virus and the bacteria.

Normal temperature is between 97° to 99° F above that would be a fever. However above 105° F can be dangerous. At 106° F there can be convulsions and at 108° F irreversible brain damage can occur.

What are the causes?
It is usually caused by bacterial or viral infections.

Additional causes for a fever are:-
A response to immunization in children,
Ear infections, bone infections, sinus infections, urinary tract infections, certain inflammatory diseases, gastroenteritis, autoimmune disorders, cancer, blood clots.
Certain medications, heat exhaustion, extreme sunburn.
A sudden change in the weather, unhygienic lifestyle.

What are the symptoms?
Shivering, chills, little or no appetite, an increased pulse rate, increased heart rate, sweating, muscle ache, joint pains, dehydration, sometimes vomiting or diarrhea, weakness, nausea, sore throat, fatigue, dizziness, headache, light-headedness, confusion and irritability.

NATURAL REMEDIES

- Drink 1 glass of water or juice every hour while awake.

- Roast dried okra seeds and grind fine. Boil ½ cup of the ground seeds in 2 glasses of water for 15 minutes. Cool and strain. Adults 1 cup, children ½ cup, babies 1 tablespoon. Take it 3 times daily after each meal.

- Steep 2 teaspoons of chamomile, rosemary or thyme, or mix them to 1 liter of boiling water for 7 minutes. Drink warm. Take 1 cup three times daily.

- Boil 1oz of crushed ginger in 1 liter of water for 15 minutes. Add 30 basil leaves to it and steep for 10 minutes. It can be sweetened with a little honey. Drink 1 cup three times daily for three days.

- Steep 1oz of sage leaves to 1 liter of boiling water for 30 minutes. Drink 4 cups daily.

- Steep 9 lemon leaves in 1 liter of boiling water for 30 minutes. Drink 4 cups daily.

- Steep the mashed rind of 1 lemon to 1 glass of boiling water for 20 minutes. Sweeten with some honey. Drink 4 cups daily.

- Blend 2 lemons with some water very well. Add 4 spoonful's of honey and enough water to make 2 liters. Strain. Drink throughout the day.

- Steep 10 neem leaves to 4 cups of boiling water for 30 minutes.
  Adults 1 cup, children ½ cup.
  Take it 4 times daily.

- Steep 4 tablespoons of crushed mint leaves to 1 liter of boiling water for 20 minutes.
  Drink 1 cup 4 times daily.

- Steep 1oz of ginger in 1 liter of boiling water for 20 minutes.
  Drink 1 cup three times daily.

- Steep 2 crushed garlic cloves in 2 cups of boiling water for 10 minutes. Strain.
  Drink 1 cup twice daily.

- Soak 1 cup of raisins in 1 liter of water for 1 hour. Crush the raisins in the water and strain the liquid. Add the juice of 1 lime to it.
  Drink 1 cup four times daily.

- Boil an apple in 2 cups of water till it gets soft. Strain the water. Add 1 tablespoon of honey to it.

- Soak 3 lettuce leaves in 3 cups of warm water for 20 minutes. Strain it. Add 1 tablespoon of honey to it. Allow it to cool.
  Drink 1 cup three times daily.

- Mix half a glass of grapefruit juice and half a glass of water.
  Take it twice daily.

- Add a pinch of cayenne powder to a cup of herbal tea.
  Drink it twice daily.

- Make a combination of cucumber, carrot and beet juice. Drink it daily.

- Have lots of citrus fruits and juices.

- Eat the soursop fruit.

- Soak a wash cloth in cool tap water, wring out the excess water.
  Sponge the armpits, feet, hands and groin.

- **Cold compress** – Dip a face towel into a basin of ice and ice water 2/3 full. Wring it making sure that it does not drip. Apply it to the forehead and the back of the neck. Change every 3 minutes for 20-30 minutes. At the end of the treatment dry the forehead very well and avoid chilling.

- Add 2 tablespoons of vinegar in a basin of cold water and use as a cold compress to the forehead, tummy and around the soles of the feet.

- Steep 1oz of red rose petals or parsley in 1 liter of boiling water for 20 minutes. Cool.
  Use it as a cold compress over the eyes. Take a rest.
  See Cold Compress method above.

- Apply an icepack over the forehead.

- Slice a potato and soak it in vinegar.
  Put it on your forehead.

- Put 3 egg whites in a bowl and beat them for 1 minute.
  Soak a thin cotton cloth in the egg white.

Place the soaked cloth on the soles of the feet. Wear socks to keep the cloth in place. When the cloths dry out and become warm, replace them with new ones.
Repeat until the fever is reduced.

- Mix 5 drops of lavender, eucalyptus, clove or tea tree oil with 1 teaspoon of coconut oil.
  Massage the temples, back of neck, top of hands and soles.

- Warm a mixture of 2 crushed garlic cloves and 2 tablespoons of olive or coconut oil.
  Apply it over the sole of each foot. Wrap your feet with gauze so that the garlic can stay in place. Leave it on overnight.

- Add 1 drop each of peppermint, eucalyptus or lavender essential oil to a cool water bath.

- Add ½ cup of vinegar to lukewarm bath water.
  Soak in it for 10 minutes.

- Add 2 tablespoons of ginger powder to a warm water bath. Soak in it for 10 minutes. Pat dry your body and rest. Cover with a blanket.

N.B. Do a patch test on the forearm before taking this bath.

- Hot foot bath.
  See the Hydrotherapy Section.

Health Tips

- Take a complete bed rest for one or two days.

- Consume plenty of green leafy vegetables.

- Drink clean water.

- Drink at least 8 – 10 glasses of water daily.

- Eat fresh food.

- Avoid eating refrigerated foods.

- Avoid smoking.

- Avoid consuming alcoholic drinks.

- Avoid consuming heavy food. Eat light.

- Avoid consuming junk food.

- Protect yourself from the ill effects of weather changes.

- Take a bath daily.

- Practice proper hygiene.

SORE THROAT

What is a sore throat?
A painful or tender throat because of an infection.

It can be due to smoke, a cold, coughing, dust, lots of talking, loud talking or singing, gum infections.

What are the causes?
Viral, bacterial, or fungal infections; tooth or gum infections; irritants like pollution, smoking, acid reflux, or dry air; excessive shouting; dust, allergic reactions; an intake of drinks and foods which are very hot.

The other causes are:-
Infection of the laryngitis, influenza, herpangina, and mumps.

What are the signs and indications?
Dry throat, difficulty in swallowing food.
Pain or an abrasive sensation in the throat.
Pain that increases while talking and eating.
Tenderness and swollen glands in the neck.
White patches or pus on the tonsils.
Bloated and red tonsils.
Croaky or subdued voice.
Swollen lymph nodes.

NATURAL REMEDIES

- Blend 1 grapefruit, 1 orange, 2 lemons, 3 garlic cloves and ½ large onion with enough water so that the mixture can turn in the blender, then add 3 drops of peppermint oil. Refrigerate and warm before serving.
  Adults 1 cup, children ½ cup daily, taken by spoonful at a time during the day.

- Blend 10 garlic cloves, 2" piece of ginger or 2 teaspoons of powdered ginger, ¼ of an onion, 1 teaspoon cayenne powder, ½ cup lemon juice and 4 cups of warm water. Sweeten with honey.
  Adults 1 cup, children ½ cup daily, taken by spoonful at a time during the day.

- **Garlic syrup**: Put one cup of finely minced garlic, one teaspoon powdered cloves and 1 ½ tablespoons grated ginger or 1 teaspoon powdered ginger in a pan. Add enough honey or molasses to cover it. Cover and simmer on low heat for about 25 minutes stirring constantly to avoid burning. A little water can be added.
  Take 1 tablespoon for adults, 1 teaspoon for children every hour.

- Boil 1oz of slippery elm bark in 1 liter of water for 20 minutes. Drink 1 warm cup twice daily.

- Steep 1 tablespoon of sage in 2 cups of boiling water for 30 minutes.
  Drink 1 cup twice daily.

- Steep 1oz of ginger in 1 liter of boiling water for 20 minutes. Drink 1 cup three times daily.

- Steep 2 teaspoons of chamomile to 1 liter of boiling water for 7 minutes. Drink warm.
  Take 1 cup three times daily.

- Steep 1oz of basil leaves in 1 liter of boiling water for 20 minutes.
  Drink 1 cup three times daily.

- Stir ¼ teaspoon of turmeric powder into a glass of warm water. Drink it slowly in the morning on an empty stomach.
  Do it for four days.

- Combine the juice of half a lemon and a little honey in a glass of hot water.
  Drink it twice daily.

- Add a pinch of turmeric to 1 cup of warm milk.
  Drink it before going to bed.

- Combine boiled water with lemon and pineapple juice.
  Freeze in an ice cube tray.
  Suck the ice cubes when necessary.

- Warm 2oz of honey and stir in 6 teaspoons of lime juice.
  When it is cool add 8 grated garlic cloves.
  Take 2 teaspoons 3 times daily.

- Add 2 tablespoons of honey to 1 cup of hot water.
  Drink it three times daily.

- Eat 1 teaspoon of honey just before bedtime.

- Combine a few drops of cinnamon oil and 1 teaspoon of honey.
  Take it twice daily.

- Chew a piece of ginger until it gets very fine, taking in the juice.

- Eat 1 raw clove of garlic.

- Have oranges, tomatoes, strawberries, squash, mangoes, and red peppers in your diet.

- Combine 1 pint of vegetable stock, 2 onions sliced thinly, 1 bay leaf, 6 cloves and salt to taste. Boil then simmer for 30 minutes. Remove the bay leaf and cloves. Serve it hot.

- Steep 1oz of sage in 1 liter of boiling water for 30 minutes.
  Gargle with it at intervals throughout the day.

- Steep 1oz of basil leaves in 1 liter of boiling water for 30 minutes.
  Gargle with it at intervals throughout the day.

- Boil 1oz of fenugreek seeds in 1 liter of water for 20 minutes.
  Gargle with it four times a day.

- Combine lemon juice with some hot water.
  Gargle with it at intervals throughout the day.

- Stir ½ teaspoon of turmeric powder and ½ teaspoon of salt in a glass of warm water.

Gargle with it twice daily.

- Steep 2 tablespoons of red rose petals or red hibiscus flowers in 2 cups of boiling water for 10 minutes.
Gargle with it at intervals throughout the day.

- Mix 1 teaspoon of salt and 1 tablespoon of apple cider vinegar in 1 cup of warm water.
Gargle with it several times a day.

- Mix ½ teaspoon of baking soda in 1 glass of warm water.
Gargle with it several times a day.

- Add a pinch of cayenne to a cup of warm water.
Gargle with it.

- Put 2 drops of clove, cinnamon or ginger oil in a glass of warm water.
Gargle with it 6 times daily.

- Salt gargle after meals.

SALT GARGLE

Procedure:

1. Put 1 teaspoon salt into 2 glasses of hot water and stir until it is melted. The water temperature should be to as hot as can be tolerated for drinking.
2. Gargle till all 2 glasses is used up.
It is best done after meals.

If the sore throat is severe with a harsh voice, it may be repeated every hour when awake. Don't drink cold drinks while the sore throat is on.

- **FIGS GARGLE**

Procedure:

Steep 2 tablespoons of dried figs in 2 glasses of water for 20 minutes. Strain and add 1 teaspoon of honey.
Gargle till all 2 glasses is used up.

- Mix one tablespoon of Garlic Oil in one pint of rubbing alcohol.
Rub it on the sides of the throat and the face.

Garlic Oil: Heat 1oz olive oil and 3 cloves of crushed garlic for about 3 minutes, strain and bottled for when ready to use. 3 drops of eucalyptus oil or glycerin can be added to help preserve it. Store in the refrigerator for when ready to use.

- Vinegar liniment.
Use this liniment to soak the cloth in for a Heating Compress For The Neck.
See the Hydrotherapy Section.

Vinegar Liniment: Mix 1 teaspoon of wintergreen oil and 2 cups of apple cider vinegar. Soak a folded cloth in it, wring out and apply it to the area.
The wintergreen will bring blood to the area and the vinegar reduces pain.
N.B. check for skin sensitivity to the wintergreen oil.

Health Tips

- Wash your hands frequently.

- Drink lots of water and fluids.

- Cough whenever you need to.

- Avoid holding the cough.

- Avoid talking too much.

- Avoid drinking cold drinks.

- Avoid dairy products.

- Avoid eating too much sweet food.

- Avoid smoking.

HYDROTHERAPY TREATMENTS

HOT FOOT BATH

It is very good for headaches, colds, flu, coughs, congestion, nosebleed, earache, sinusitis, menstrual pains, fatigue, fever, pelvic cramps and congestion, prostate disorders, nervous tension, toothaches, backaches, infections, relaxation, stimulates circulation and warms the body.

Items needed:

1 bucket about quarter filled with hot water.
Small basin of ice water.
Large pan of very hot water.
2 washcloths for the head compress.
1 sheet and a blanket or 2 sheets.
1 hand towel for the neck.
1 bath towel.
1 bath mat.

Procedure:

1.　　Drape a blanket to completely cover a chair, then cover the blanket with a sheet.

2.　　Place a bucket ¼ filled with hot water on a bath mat in front of the chair.

3.　　Remove clothing, sit and wrap with the sheet, then the blanket.

4. Close all doors and windows.

5. Place the feet into the bucket and wrap the sheet and blanket around the bucket to avoid the circulation of air.

6. Wrap a hand towel around the neck to hold the sheet and blanket in place.

7. Apply a cold compress to the forehead, changing it every 3 minutes.

8. Maintain the water temperature in the bucket by adding more hot water continuously by pushing the persons feet to one side and placing your hands as a shield between the feet and the flow of hot water.

9. Continue adding the hot water for 20-30 minutes or an hour if needed. When sweating begins give the person water to drink at intervals throughout the treatment.

10. At the end of the treatment lift the feet up and pour cold water over them very quickly, dry and put on warm socks. Unwrap and dry the body. Dress, cover warmly and rest for 30-60 minutes. Take a cool shower.

A heating pad placed on the lower abdomen and upper thighs or a heating compress on the feet repeated every 4 hours can be used to replace the hot foot bath.

N.B. Do not use this treatment for persons with diabetes, loss of feelings, unconscious, arteriosclerosis, elevated pulse.

STEAM INHALATION

Effects:

1.   Relieves nasal and lung congestions.

2.   Relieves coughs.

3.   Secretions are loosen and it is easier to expectorate.

4.   Blood flow is increased to the throat and lungs.

5.   Relieves sinus headaches.

Contraindications:

1.   Persons suffering with congestive heart failure.

2.   Persons suffering with asthma.

Items needed:

Basin with boiling water
Umbrella and sheet
Bedside stand and chair
A few drops of wintergreen or eucalyptus oil, or
1 teaspoon Vicks VapoRub, or 2 tablespoons of herbs.

Procedure:

1.   Fill a face basin with boiling water and add medication or herb if desired.

2. Put it on a table or bedside stand. Sit on a chair and open an umbrella over the head then cover with a sheet to form a tent over the head and basin. Instead of the umbrella and sheet, a large thick towel can be used to cover the head and basin.

3. Inhale the steam for 30 to 60 minutes 2 – 3 times daily.

4. Dry the face and any other moist areas of the body.

5. Rest for half an hour.

HOT SWEAT BATH

Procedure:

1. Sit in a hot tub of water for 20 minutes until sweating is in abundance.

2. Dry quickly. Rest and cover warmly.

3. Have a hot drink of weak unsweetened lemonade.

4. After one hour of sweating do a quick rubbing alcohol sponge or rub with a cold washcloth.
   Change the clothing and rest again for another hour if possible.

HEATING COMPRESS FOR THE NECK

Method:

1. Cut a strip of cotton about 2 x 14 inches or long enough to wrap around the neck. Soak it in cold water and squeeze it loosely, applying it to the skin surface.

2. Cover with a piece of plastic 3 x 14 inches making sure that it completely covers the cotton strip.

3. Wrap a scarf or large wool sock around the throat over the cotton and plastic to cover them, pin it securely in place with safety pins.

4. Take care that the compress is not too tight to interfere with the circulation. It can be left on for several hours or it is best applied at night and removed in the morning until relief is obtained.

5. Remove the compress and rub the area with a cold cloth. Dry thoroughly.

Other Book Titles by the Same Author

Can be viewed at this link:
http://www.amazon.com/author/monicasidoine

Home Remedies For Cancer

Home Remedies For Losing Weight

Home Remedies For Blood Pressure and Diabetes

Home Remedies For Headaches and Insomnia

Home Remedies For Sinusitis and Tonsillitis

Home Remedies For Constipation and Diarrhea

Home Remedies For Asthma and Bronchitis

Home Remedies For Dehydration and Vomiting

Home Remedies For Pneumonia and Tuberculosis

Home Remedies For Stress, Depression and Anxiety

Home Remedies For Heart Attack and Strokes

NOTES

NOTES

NOTES

NOTES

NOTES